FOOD FOR THOUGHT

Biblical Truths They Never Taught Us

VOLUME 1

God's Original Diet and the Healing of the Nations

Rev. Duane A. Quamina

Food For Thought

Published in the United States by **Quamina Legacy Press**
First Edition: 2026

Paperback ISBN: 979-8-9957271-0-1
eBook ISBN: 979-8-9957271-1-8

Library of Congress Control Number: 2026909827

Cover Design: **Quamina Legacy Press**
Printed in the United States of America

Permissions:
Readers, teachers, and institutions may share or teach from this text for the upliftment of humanity. Do not distort its message or weaponize its teachings to harm others.

Scripture Notice:
All Scripture quotations are from the King James Version (KJV), unless otherwise noted.

Author: Unknown

Inquiries:
Quamina Legacy Press
2230 Route 70 W, STE 2 #1084
Cherry Hill, NJ 08002
info@quaminalegacypress.com | 215-651-0229

All Glory to God Alone

Table Of Contents

PREFACE
WHAT I SAW, WHAT I FELT, WHAT I NOW UNDERSTAND

On one Resurrection Sunday, after church service, I attended a gathering filled with gospel music, fellowship, and celebration. There were at least ten gospel groups. The room was alive with praise—but something else was present too.

I began to observe.

Many of the people—good people, faithful people—were struggling physically:

- Walking with canes
- Breathing heavily
- Speaking openly about recent health scares
- Sharing testimonies of near-death experiences

I noticed something else. The food that was served that day. Everything had meat in it.

There were no options aligned with how I now live. I could not eat. But more than that—I could not ignore what I was seeing.

People were eating, but they were not well.

And in that moment, I felt something deeper than concern.

I felt grief.

Not because they were doing something wrong—but because **they did not know**.

A Memory That Came Back

I was reminded of my uncle William Henry. He was a good man. Quite handsome and a military veteran.

He suffered from congestive heart failure. I watched as my mother—out of love for her brother—continued to feed him the very foods that were contributing to his condition.

And I said nothing.

Not because I didn't care… but because I didn't know.

She didn't know either.

And that's how cycles continue—not through harm, but through **lack of knowledge**.

A Personal Transformation

As an athlete, my life changed when I removed animal products from my diet.

- My energy improved
- My endurance increased
- My recovery accelerated

What I experienced physically… I later began to understand spiritually and scientifically.

The data confirmed what my body already knew.

Why This Book Exists

This book is not written to judge.

It is written to **share**.

To place scripture, observation, and evidence side by side and ask:

Have we drifted from what God originally gave us?

If so…

Can returning to that design restore not only our health—but our lives?

Amen.

SCRIPTURAL EPIGRAPH

GENESIS 1:29 (KJV)

"And God said, Behold, I have given you every herb bearing seed, which is upon the face of all the earth, and every tree, in the which is the fruit of a tree yielding seed; to you it shall be for meat."

CHAPTER 1
THE ORIGINAL COMMAND

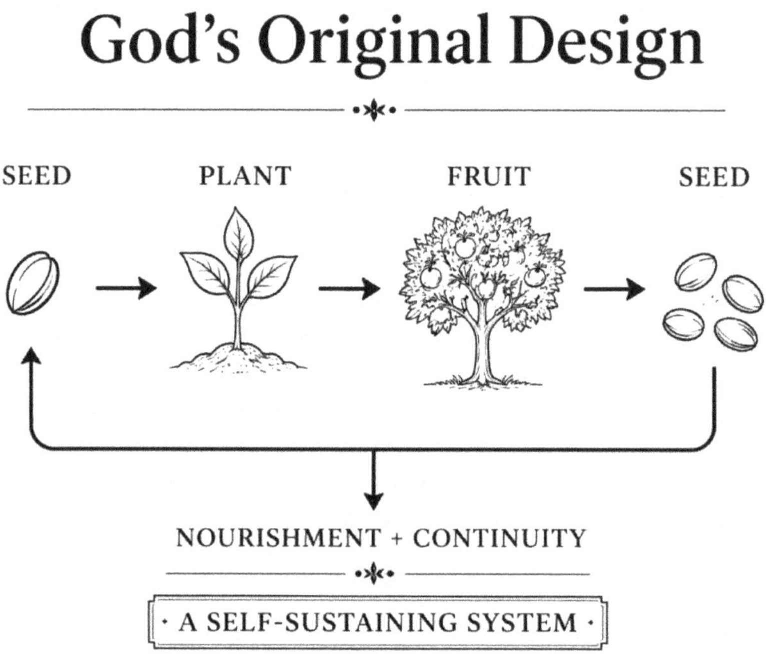

In a world filled with conflicting information about diet, health, and longevity, it is easy to overlook a simple truth: humanity was not left without instruction.

From the very beginning, before disease, before death, before confusion—God spoke clearly about what sustains life.

GENESIS 1:29 (KJV)
"And God said, Behold, I have given you every herb bearing seed, which is upon the face of all the earth, and every tree, in the which is the fruit of a tree yielding seed; to you it shall be for meat."

This was not a suggestion. It was not a cultural norm. It was a **divine provision**.

God did not create man and then leave him to discover how to survive. He created both **man and his food source simultaneously**, ensuring that life would be sustained through a system that was complete, regenerative, and self-perpetuating.

Notice the specificity:

- **Every herb bearing seed**
- **Every tree with fruit yielding seed**

This is not random. This is design.

Seed-bearing plants represent more than food—they represent **continuity**. Every meal contains within it the capacity to reproduce itself. This is a system of **"life producing life, not death producing sustenance."**

There is no mention of killing.

There is no mention of blood.

There is no mention of disease management.

Only provision.

Only abundance.

Only life.

A System Without Sickness

Before the fall, there is no record of disease. No hospitals. No medications. No interventions.

Why?

Because the system was aligned.

Food was not only nourishment—it was **protection**.

Modern science is only now catching up to what was established in the beginning: that whole, plant-based foods contain the nutrients, antioxidants, fiber, and compounds necessary to sustain and protect the human body.

But in Genesis, this was not "discovered." It was **given**.

The Misunderstood Word "Meat"

In the King James Version, the word "meat" appears in Genesis 1:29. However, in its original usage, "meat" simply means **food**—not specifically animal flesh.

This distinction is critical.

What God defined as food in the beginning was not animal-based. It was **plant-based, seed-bearing, and life-sustaining**.

The Pattern Established

Genesis 1:29 establishes a pattern that echoes throughout scripture:

- God provides **plants for food**
- God provides **trees for healing**
- God designs a system that requires no destruction to sustain life

This pattern is not isolated. It is reinforced later in scripture, pointing us back to the same truth.

CHAPTER 2
HEALING BUILT INTO CREATION

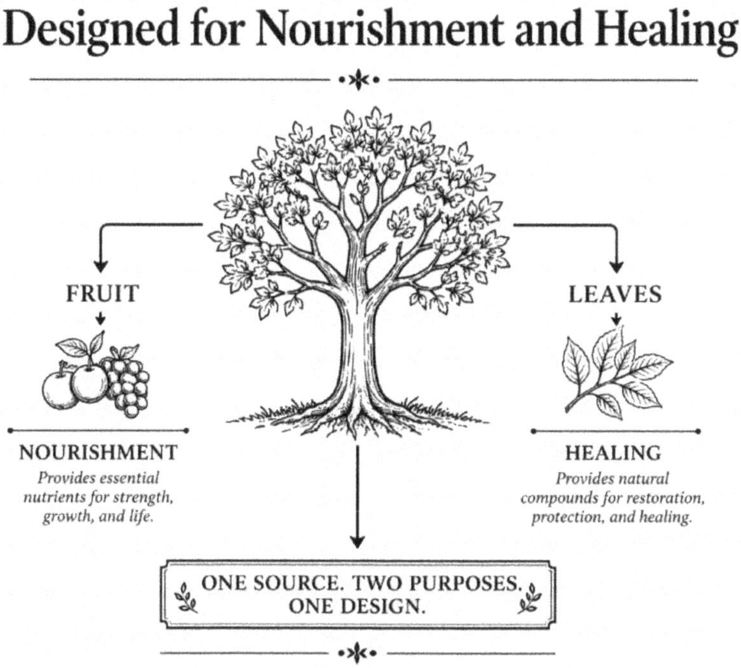

If Genesis introduces us to God's provision, later scriptures reveal something even deeper:

That provision was not only for nourishment—but for healing.

EZEKIEL 47:12 (KJV)
"And by the river upon the bank thereof… shall grow all trees for meat… the fruit thereof shall be for meat, and the leaf thereof for medicine."

Here we see a continuation of the same system:
- Trees for food
- Leaves for medicine

This is not a new concept—it is a **reaffirmation**.

God did not create a separate system for healing. Healing was already embedded within the system of food itself.

Food as Medicine — Not a Modern Idea

Today, the phrase "food as medicine" is widely discussed in health circles. But this is not a modern discovery—it is an ancient truth.

The prophet Ezekiel reveals that the same trees that provide nourishment also provide **healing**.

There is no division between the two.

In God's system:

- What you eat sustains you
- What you eat heals you

The Final Confirmation

This truth does not end in the Old Testament. It carries through to the final book of the Bible.

REVELATION 22:2 (KJV)
"In the midst of the street of it... was there the tree of life... and the leaves of the tree were for the healing of the nations." —

At the end of scripture, we return to the beginning.

The Tree of Life appears again—not as a relic of the past, but as a **promise for the future**.

And what does it provide?

- Fruit for sustenance
- Leaves for healing

The same pattern.

From Genesis… to Ezekiel… to Revelation…

God never changed the design.

A System We Drifted From

If God's system includes both nourishment and healing within plant life, then we must ask a difficult but necessary question:

What happens when we move away from that system?

Do we lose access to the very mechanisms designed to sustain and repair the body?

Do we replace a system of prevention with a system of reaction?

These are not questions of condemnation—but of reflection.

Returning to What Was Given

The scriptures do not force—they reveal.

They do not condemn—they invite.

The invitation is simple:

To reconsider what was given in the beginning…

And to ask whether the path forward may actually be a return.

CHAPTER 3
THE FLOOD AND THE SHIFT

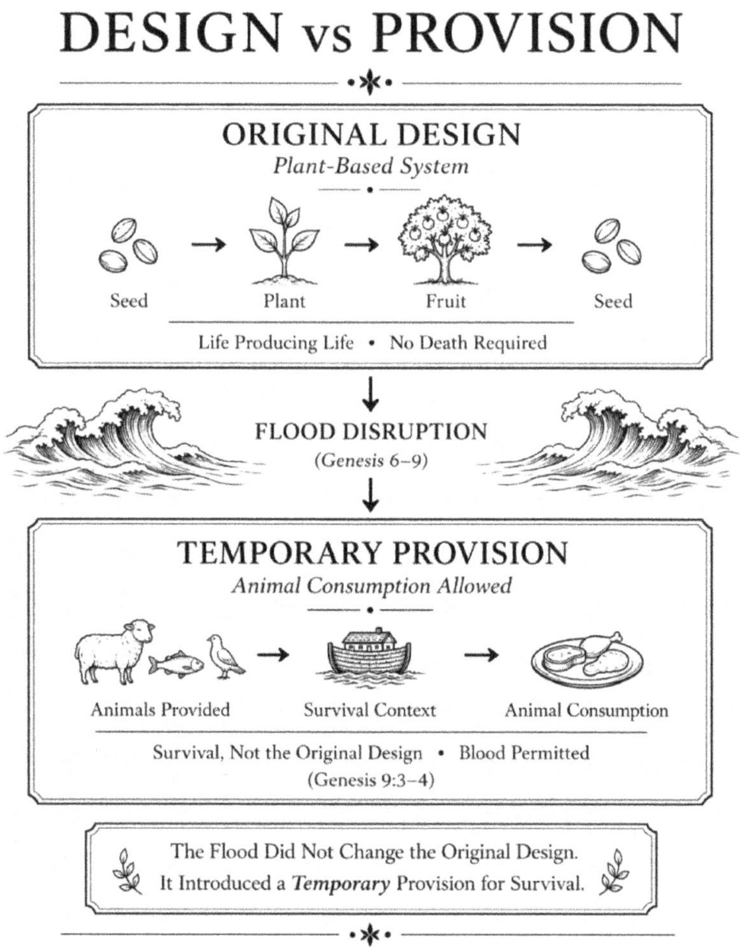

To understand where we are today, we must first understand **what changed**.

Genesis 1:29 (KJV)
established God's original design: a plant-based, life-sustaining system. But later in scripture, we encounter what appears to be a significant shift.

Genesis 9:3 (KJV)
"Every moving thing that liveth shall be meat for you; even as the green herb have I given you all things."

At first glance, this seems like a permanent expansion of the human diet. But context matters.

A World After Collapse

The flood described in Genesis was not just a judgment—it was an **environmental reset**.

- Vegetation was destroyed
- Agricultural systems were disrupted
- The earth's natural food supply was temporarily compromised

In that context, God made a provision:

"Every moving thing… shall be food for you."

This was not the introduction of a new ideal—it was a **response to a broken environment**.

Provision vs. Design

There is a difference between:

- **What God allows**
- **What God originally designed**

Genesis 1 reflects **perfection**

Genesis 9 reflects **adaptation**

This distinction is critical.

Because what is permitted in a moment of survival is not always what is intended for long-term thriving.

"Even As the Green Herb" — A Clue Often Overlooked

Notice the phrase:

"Even as the green herb have I given you all things."

This suggests continuity, not replacement.

It does not say:

"Instead of plants..."

It says:

"Just as I gave you plants..."

Meaning:

- The original system was still valid
- The new provision was **added**, not substituted

A Temporary Permission in a Fallen World

After the flood:

- The world was no longer in its original state
- Humanity was no longer operating in perfect alignment
- Survival required flexibility

But as vegetation returned... as the earth recovered... the question remains:

Were we meant to stay in survival mode?

Or return to the system God declared "very good"?

Patterns of Permission in Scripture

Throughout the Bible, we see a pattern:

God allows certain things—not because they are ideal, but because humanity is not yet ready to fully align.

Examples include:

- Kings in Israel
- Divorce laws
- Dietary expansions

These were not always expressions of perfection—but accommodations within imperfection.

The Cost of the Shift

When diet shifts from plant-based to animal-based, something changes at a foundational level:

- Life is no longer sustained purely by regenerative systems
- Death becomes part of sustenance
- The body begins processing substances it was not originally designed to rely on

This introduces new variables:

- Cholesterol
- Saturated fat
- Inflammatory compounds

These are not abstract concepts—they are measurable realities.

And over time, they manifest as disease.

A Question for Reflection

If God's original system required no killing…

And the later system introduced it under crisis…

Then we must ask:

Which system leads to life… and which one sustains us in survival?

CHAPTER 4
THE MODERN DIET AND THE EVIDENCE OF DISEASE

We now move from scripture to observation.

Because truth is not only written—it is **demonstrated**.

If a system is aligned with life, it should produce life.

If it is not, the evidence will reveal itself.

The State of Health in Modern Society

According to the Centers for Disease Control and Prevention:

- Heart disease is the **leading cause of death in the United States**
- One person dies every 33 seconds from cardiovascular disease
- High LDL cholesterol is a **primary contributing factor**

This is not rare.

This is not isolated.

This is **systemic**.

What Drives Heart Disease?

The buildup of LDL cholesterol—often referred to as "bad cholesterol"—is strongly associated with:

- Diets high in animal products
- Saturated fat intake
- Processed meats

Over time, this leads to:

- Plaque buildup in arteries
- Reduced blood flow
- Increased risk of heart attack and stroke

This is not theory. This is established science.

Harvard's Findings

Research from the Harvard T.H. Chan School of Public Health consistently shows:

- High consumption of red and processed meats is linked to:
    - Heart disease
    - Type 2 diabetes
    - Certain cancers

- Diets rich in plant-based foods are associated with:
    - Lower mortality rates
    - Improved cardiovascular health
    - Reduced chronic disease risk

NIH Research

The National Institutes of Health has documented that:

- Whole-food, plant-based diets can:
    - Lower LDL cholesterol significantly
    - Reduce inflammation
    - Improve insulin sensitivity

In some cases, these diets have been shown to:

- **Reverse early-stage heart disease**
- Reduce reliance on medication

The Blue Zones — Living Proof

Studies of Blue Zones—regions where people live the longest—reveal a consistent pattern:

- Diets are primarily plant-based
- Animal products are minimal or occasional
- Whole, unprocessed foods dominate

These populations experience:

- Lower rates of heart disease
- Lower rates of cancer
- Greater longevity

The Pattern Becomes Clear

When we align the data with scripture, something remarkable emerges:

Scripture	Modern Evidence
Plants for food (**Genesis 1:29 (KJV)**)	Plant diets reduce disease
Leaves for healing (**Ezekiel 47:12 (KJV)**)	Plants contain healing compounds
Tree of Life restores (**Revelation 22:2 (KJV)**)	Plant-based living increases longevity

The pattern is consistent across both domains.

Managing Disease vs Preventing It

Modern medicine often focuses on:

- Treating symptoms
- Managing chronic conditions
- Prescribing medication

But rarely asks:

What caused the condition in the first place?

When diet is the root cause, medication becomes:

- A temporary solution
- A long-term dependency

A System Worth Reexamining

We are now faced with a reality that cannot be ignored:

- The current dietary system is producing disease at scale
- The original system described in scripture promotes life

"This is not coincidence. This is contrast."

Diet Type	Outcome
Plant-Based	Lower cholesterol, lower disease
Animal-Based	Higher cholesterol, higher disease

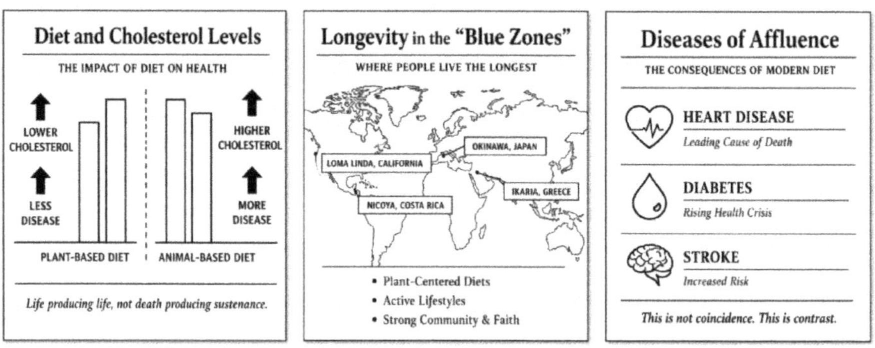

Figure 1 — Diet, Disease, and Longevity

FOOD FOR THOUGHT: CHARTS (DROP-IN)

Research. Scripture. A Path to Healing.

CHART 1: DIET & CHOLESTEROL IMPACT

The Evidence Is Clear.

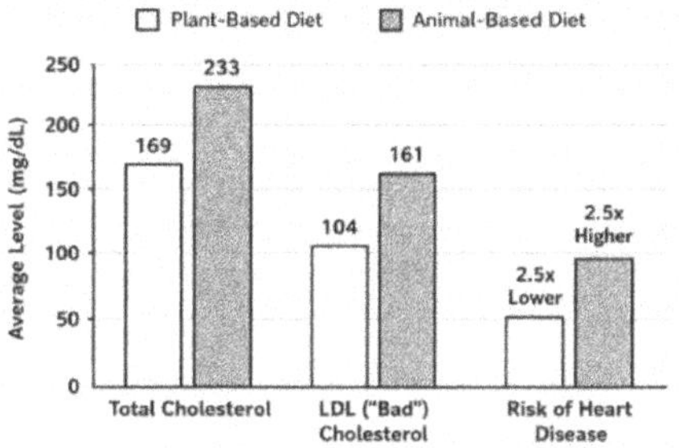

Studies show plant-based diets lower cholesterol and reduce the risk of heart disease.

Source: Ornish D., et al. JAMA. 1990; Esselstyn C., et al. Am J Cardiol. 2014.

CHART 2: BLUE ZONES LONGEVITY COMPARISON

Plant-Rich People. Longer Lives.

Blue Zone Region	Primary Diet (Predominant)	Life Expectancy (Average)	Key Lifestyle Factor
Okinawa (Japan)	Vegetables, fruits, soy, whole grains	87 years	Plant-based, active, strong community
Sardinia (Italy)	Beans, whole grains, vegetables, nuts	86 years	Plant-rich, family, purpose
Loma Linda (California, USA)	Fruits, vegetables, whole grains, nuts	85 years (Adventists)	Plant-based, faith, moderation
Ikaria (Greece)	Vegetables, legumes, olive oil, nuts	90 years	Plant-rich, rest, strong relationships
Nicoya Peninsula (Costa Rica)	Beans, corn, fruits, vegetables	88 years	Plant-based, hard work, community

Common Thread: Mostly plants. Stronger lives.

Source: Dan Buettner, The Blue Zones (National Geographic, 2008).

CHART 3: DIET & DISEASE RISK COMPARISON

What We Eat Shapes How We Live.

Health Condition	Plant-Based Diet (Risk)	Animal-Based Diet (Risk)	Difference	What the Research Shows
Heart Disease	Up to 73% Lower	Higher	Up to 73% Reduction	Plant-based diets are associated with significantly lower heart disease risk.
Type 2 Diabetes	Up to 62% Lower	Higher	Up to 62% Reduction	Plant-based diets improve blood sugar control and reduce diabetes risk.
Obesity	Lower	Higher	Significant Reduction	Plant-based diets are linked to healthy weight and lower obesity rates.
Certain Cancers	Up to 40% Lower	Higher	Up to 40% Reduction	Plant-rich diets may lower risk of colon, breast, and prostate cancers.
Overall Mortality	Up to 25% Lower	Higher	Up to 25% Reduction	Plant-based diets are linked to longer life and lower death rates.

Food is not just fuel. It is information. It can protect. Or it can harm.

Sources: American Journal of Clinical Nutrition, 2021 | Harvard T.H. Chan School of Public Health, 2019 | Adventist Health Studies.

GOD'S ORIGINAL DESIGN. OUR HEALTHY FUTURE.

"And God said, Behold, I have given you every herb bearing seed... to you it shall be for meat."

— GENESIS 1:29 (NKJV)

HOW TO USE THESE CHARTS:

- Copy and paste into your Word document
- Resize as needed
- Great for teaching, presentations, and handouts
- Designed to support truth with evidence

All Glory to God Alone. | Quamina Legacy Press | www.quaminalegacypress.com

Figure 2 — Research Comparison Charts

The body does not lie. The pattern reveals the truth. Plant-based dietary patterns consistently correlate with lower disease risk and longer life expectancy across global populations.

CHAPTER 5
THE TWO TREES REVISITED

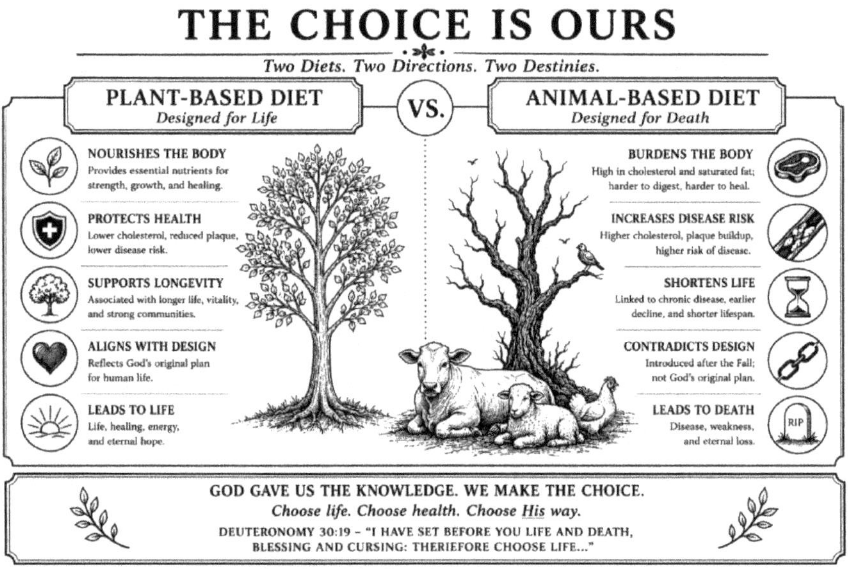

In the opening chapters of scripture, we are introduced to one of the most profound moments in human history: the presence of two trees in the Garden of Eden.

- The **Tree of Life**
- The **Tree of the Knowledge of Good and Evil**

Most discussions focus on disobedience. Few pause to examine **what these trees represent beyond the surface**.

The Tree of Life — A System of Healing

Scripture gives us clarity about the Tree of Life—not in Genesis alone, but in its final appearance.

REVELATION 22:2 (KJV)
"…the tree of life… and the leaves of the tree were for the healing of the nations."

This aligns perfectly with what we saw earlier:

- Trees provide food
- Leaves provide healing

The Tree of Life is not merely symbolic—it represents a **sustaining, healing system rooted in creation itself**.

The Tree of Knowledge — A Deeper Question

Now we turn to the second tree.

GENESIS 2:17 (KJV)
"...of the tree of the knowledge of good and evil, thou shalt not eat of it..."

This command is direct:

Do not eat.

But why?

Traditionally, this is interpreted as a moral test. And that interpretation holds weight.

But scripture often carries layers—surface meaning and deeper reflection.

Let us explore, carefully and respectfully, an additional perspective.

Awareness of Life and Death

Animals possess awareness.

- They recognize threat
- They respond to intent
- They distinguish between safety and danger

Approach an animal gently—it receives you.

Approach it with harm—it resists, sometimes violently.

There is an awareness present.

A knowing.

A distinction between **good and evil... life and death**.

A Thought for Reflection (Not Doctrine)

What if the command "do not eat" carries a deeper implication?

Not a contradiction of scripture—but a layer of reflection within it.

Could it be that consuming life that is aware of its own destruction introduces humanity into a different relationship with creation?

A relationship no longer based purely on sustaining life...

But involving the taking of it.

This is not a declaration.

It is a question.

Why This Matters

Because the act of eating is not just physical—it is **spiritual, emotional, and systemic**.

When the source of food changes:

- The relationship to life changes
- The body processes different substances
- The system of sustenance shifts

This aligns with what we explored:

- Genesis 1 — Life sustained without death
- Genesis 9 — Life sustained through death (under condition)

Biblical Symbolism Reinforced

In Daniel 4, we see a vision of a great tree:

- It provides shelter
- It sustains animals
- Birds dwell in its branches

The tree represents a kingdom—but notice the system:

The animals live within the tree's provision. They are not the provision.

This reinforces the pattern:

- Life is sustained through what grows
- Not through what is destroyed

Returning to the Question

If one tree represents healing and life...

And the other represents knowledge tied to consequence...

Then the command becomes more than restriction—it becomes **protection**.

Protection from entering a system where:

- Death becomes normalized
- The body adapts to what it was not originally designed to rely on
- The consequences unfold over time

Holding the Tension with Wisdom

"This perspective is presented as a reflective lens, not a replacement for established doctrine."

Each reader must consider:

- What aligns with scripture
- What aligns with observable reality
- What aligns with the condition of the human body today

Because truth does not fear examination.

CHAPTER 6
DEPENDENCY VS DISCIPLINE

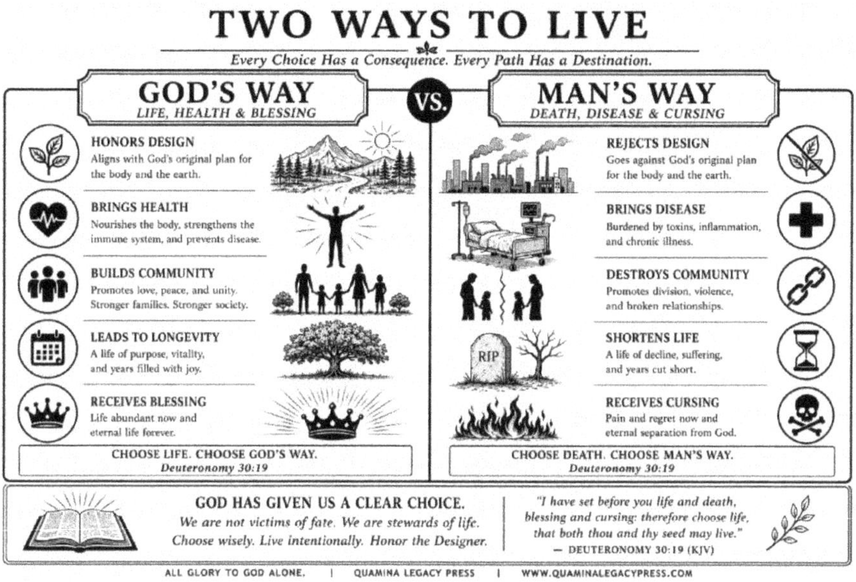

We now arrive at one of the most practical implications of this discussion.

Not theory. Not symbolism.

Reality.

The Modern Cycle

In today's world, a pattern has emerged:

1. Consume foods that contribute to disease
2. Develop chronic conditions
3. Rely on medication to manage symptoms

This cycle repeats—often for a lifetime.

A System of Management, Not Resolution

Modern medicine has achieved incredible advancements. It saves lives. It stabilizes conditions.

But in many cases, it operates within a framework of:

- **Management over elimination**
- **Treatment over prevention**

For example:

- High cholesterol → prescribed medication
- High blood pressure → prescribed medication
- Type 2 diabetes → managed long-term

But rarely is the foundational question addressed:

What created the condition?

Diet as a Root Cause

As established in Chapter 4:

- Diets high in animal products are strongly linked to chronic disease
- Plant-based diets reduce or reverse many of these conditions

This places diet not at the edge of the conversation—but at the **center of it**.

The Cost of Ignoring the Root

When the root cause is not addressed:

- Medication becomes permanent
- Side effects accumulate
- Dependency increases

This is not healing.

This is **maintenance of imbalance**.

God's System vs Man's System

Let us contrast the two:

God's Design	Modern Pattern
Prevention	Treatment
Food as medicine	Medicine as necessity
Alignment	Correction
Sustainability	Dependency

The Role of Discipline

Returning to alignment requires something that cannot be prescribed:

Discipline.

- Choosing differently
- Eating intentionally
- Breaking inherited habits

This is not always easy.

But it is necessary.

A Temple, Not a Testing Ground

Scripture reminds us:

1 Corinthians 6:19 (KJV)
"Know ye not that your body is the temple of the Holy Ghost…?"

A temple is not neglected.

It is maintained with care, intention, and respect.

What we put into the body is not trivial—it is foundational.

Breaking the Cycle

The shift begins with awareness:

- Understanding what fuels disease
- Recognizing what supports healing
- Making decisions aligned with life

This is not about perfection.

It is about **direction**.

A Return to Responsibility

We cannot control everything.

But we can control:

- What we eat
- What we learn
- What we choose moving forward

And sometimes, the most powerful change is not found in something new…

But in returning to what was given from the beginning.

CHAPTER 7
RETURNING TO THE GARDEN

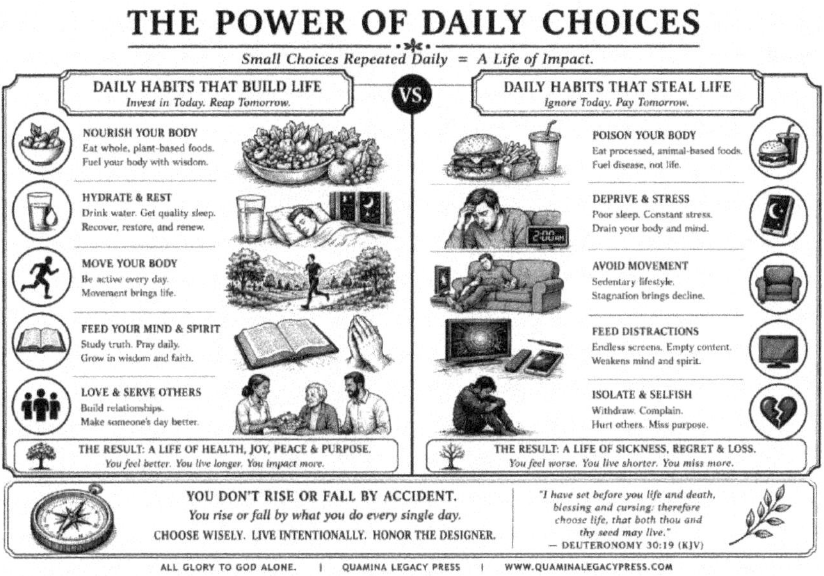

After examining scripture, history, and modern evidence, we arrive at a simple but powerful truth:

The path forward may actually be a return.

Not Backward—But Restorative

Returning to the Garden does not mean rejecting progress.

It means:

- Reclaiming alignment
- Restoring balance
- Reconnecting with design

It is not about living in the past.

It is about bringing truth forward.

What Returning Looks Like

This is not an all-or-nothing transformation. It is a process.

It begins with awareness… and continues with action.

1. Increase What Gives Life

- Fruits
- Vegetables
- Whole grains
- Nuts and seeds

These are the foods originally given.
They carry:

- Fiber
- Antioxidants
- Healing compounds

2. Reduce What Contributes to Disease

- Processed meats
- High-fat animal products
- Excessive cholesterol intake

This is not about condemnation.

It is about **recognition**.

3. Eat With Intention

Every meal becomes a decision:

- Does this support life?
- Or does this sustain imbalance?

4. Relearn What We Were Never Taught

Many of us were never educated on:

- Nutrition
- Food systems
- The connection between diet and disease

This is not accidental.

But it can be corrected.

A Shift in Mindset
We must move from:

- Convenience → Consciousness
- Habit → Intentionality
- Reaction → Prevention

Small Changes, Significant Impact

Even gradual shifts can lead to measurable outcomes:

- Lower cholesterol
- Reduced inflammation
- Improved energy
- Better long-term health

The body responds to alignment.

This Is Not About Perfection—it is about direction.

Every step toward what sustains life… matters.

CONCLUSION
HEALING THE NATIONS BEGINS WITH THE TABLE

From Genesis to Revelation, a consistent pattern emerges:

- God provides plants for food
- God provides leaves for healing
- God establishes a system rooted in life

Over time, humanity adapted.

But adaptation is not always alignment.

The Evidence Speaks

- Modern disease patterns reflect dietary choices
- Scientific research supports plant-based living
- Scripture consistently points to the same system

This is not coincidence.

It is confirmation.

A Personal Responsibility

Each of us must decide:

- What we will accept
- What we will question
- What we will change

Not out of fear... but out of understanding.

A Collective Opportunity

If individuals begin to shift:

- Families change
- Communities change
- Outcomes change

Healing does not begin in hospitals.

It begins with **daily decisions**.

The Final Thought

The same God who created life… also defined what sustains it.

Perhaps the healing we seek is not hidden.

Perhaps it has been with us from the beginning.

Closing Reflection

This book is not an ending.
It is an invitation.
To think.
To reflect.
To reconsider.
And if necessary…
To return.

The question is no longer what we were told… but what was given.

SCIENCE-BACKED FOODS FOR THE WHOLE BODY

God's original design for food was not only to sustain life—but to heal it. Modern science now confirms what was given in the beginning.

- ➔ **Brain & Cognitive Function**
  Berries, walnuts, flaxseed — support memory, focus, and neurological health.
- ➔ **Heart & Circulation**
  Leafy greens, oats, berries — help reduce cholesterol and support cardiovascular strength.
- ➔ **Liver & Detoxification**
  Beets, turmeric, garlic — assist the body in cleansing and restoring liver function.
- ➔ **Digestive System**
  Apples, ginger, chia seeds — promote healthy digestion and gut balance.
- ➔ **Bones & Structure**
  Kale, broccoli, almonds — provide essential minerals for strength and stability.
- ➔ **Immune System**
  Garlic, citrus fruits, ginger — strengthen the body's natural defenses.
- ➔ **Inflammation & Joint Health**
  Pineapple, berries, turmeric — reduce inflammation and support mobility.
- ➔ **Circulation & Blood Flow**
  Avocados, beans, pomegranates — promote healthy blood vessels and oxygen flow.

Understanding without application leaves transformation unfinished.

PRACTICAL APPLICATION — FOODS THAT HEAL

Search online for whole-food, plant-based recipes and discover simple, life-changing meals that align with God's original design.

- The journey does not end with knowledge—it begins with action.
- What you eat daily will determine what your body becomes over time.
- Below are a few clean, plant-based, practical recipes to get started.

1. Brain & Cognitive Function
Berry Brain Boost Smoothie
Ingredients:

- 1 cup blueberries (fresh or frozen)
- 1 tbsp ground flaxseed
- 1 tbsp walnuts
- 1 banana
- 1 cup almond milk

Instructions:
Blend until smooth.
Why it works:

- Berries → antioxidants for brain protection
- Flaxseed → omega-3 support
- Walnuts → cognitive function

2. Heart & Circulation
Oat & Berry Heart Bowl
Ingredients:

- 1 cup oats
- 1 cup water or almond milk
- ½ cup strawberries or blueberries
- 1 tbsp chia seeds
- 1 tsp cinnamon

Instructions:
Cook oats → top with berries, chia, cinnamon.

Why it works:

- Oats → lowers LDL cholesterol
- Berries → heart protection
- Chia → omega-3 + fiber

3. Liver Detox
Beet & Citrus Cleanse Juice
Ingredients:

- 1 beet
- 1 carrot
- 1 orange
- ½ lemon
- Small piece of ginger

Instructions:
Juice or blend + strain.
Why it works:

- Beets → liver cleansing
- Citrus → detox support
- Ginger → anti-inflammatory

4. Digestion
Apple Ginger Digestive Tonic
Ingredients:

- 1 apple
- 1 tsp grated ginger
- 1 tbsp chia seeds
- 1 cup water

Instructions:
Blend and let sit 5–10 minutes.
Why it works:

- Apple → fiber
- Ginger → gut stimulation
- Chia → digestive support

5. Bones & Structure
Green Strength Salad
Ingredients:

- Kale
- Broccoli (lightly steamed)

- Almonds
- Olive oil
- Lemon juice

Instructions:
Mix + massage kale + drizzle dressing.
Why it works:

- Kale → calcium
- Broccoli → bone density
- Almonds → minerals

6. Immune System
Garlic Ginger Immunity Soup
Ingredients:

- 3 cloves garlic
- 1 tbsp ginger
- 2 cups vegetable broth
- Carrots + celery
- Spinach

Instructions:
Simmer 15–20 minutes.
Why it works:

- Garlic → antimicrobial
- Ginger → immune support
- Greens → nutrient density

7. Inflammation & Joint Health
Turmeric Pineapple Anti-Inflammation Smoothie
Ingredients:

- 1 cup pineapple
- ½ tsp turmeric
- 1 banana
- 1 cup coconut water
- Pinch black pepper

Instructions:
Blend.
Why it works:

- Turmeric → anti-inflammatory
- Pineapple → bromelain (joint support)

8. Circulation & Blood Flow
Avocado Bean Power Bowl
Ingredients:

- Black beans
- Avocado
- Brown rice or quinoa
- Cherry tomatoes
- Lime juice

Instructions:
Layer + mix.
Why it works:

- Beans → fiber + blood sugar control
- Avocado → healthy fats
- Lime → circulation boost

Disclaimer: The material in this book is for educational purposes only. Consult your physician before making dietary or health changes.

REFLECTION & DISCUSSION QUESTIONS

- What did Genesis 1:29 (KJV) reveal to you about God's original design for food?
- How does your current diet align with what is described in scripture?
- What changes, if any, do you feel led to make after reading this book?
- What stood out to you most in the scientific evidence presented?
- How do you view the connection between food, health, and spiritual responsibility?
- In what ways can this message be shared within your family or community?
- What barriers might prevent you from making changes, and how can they be addressed?

Notes:

KEY SCRIPTURES FOR CONTINUED STUDY

GENESIS 1:29 (KJV)
"And God said, Behold, I have given you every herb bearing seed, which is upon the face of all the earth, and every tree, in the which is the fruit of a tree yielding seed; to you it shall be for meat."

GENESIS 9:3 (KJV)
"Every moving thing that liveth shall be meat for you; even as the green herb have I given you all things."

EZEKIEL 47:12 (KJV)
And by the river upon the bank thereof, on this side and on that side, shall grow all trees for meat, whose leaf shall not fade, neither shall the fruit thereof be consumed: it shall bring forth new fruit according to his months, because their waters they issued out of the sanctuary: and the fruit thereof shall be for meat, and the leaf thereof for medicine."

REVELATION 22:2 (KJV)
" In the midst of the street of it, and on either side of the river, was there the tree of life, which bare twelve manner of fruits, and yielded her fruit every month: and the leaves of the tree were for the healing of the nations."

1 CORINTHIANS 6:19 (KJV)
"What? know ye not that your body is the temple of the Holy Ghost which is in you, which ye have of God, and ye are not your own?"

AUTHOR'S CLOSING NOTE

A Personal Word to the Reader

This book was not written from a place of judgment, but from a place of realization.

There was a time when I did not know what I now understand. I watched people I loved suffer, and I did not yet have the knowledge to connect the dots.

What you have read is not meant to overwhelm you. It is meant to awaken you.

You do not have to change everything at once.

But you can begin.

One decision. One meal. One step toward alignment.

If this book has caused you to think differently, then it has done its job.

The rest is in your hands.

Amen.

ABOUT THE AUTHOR

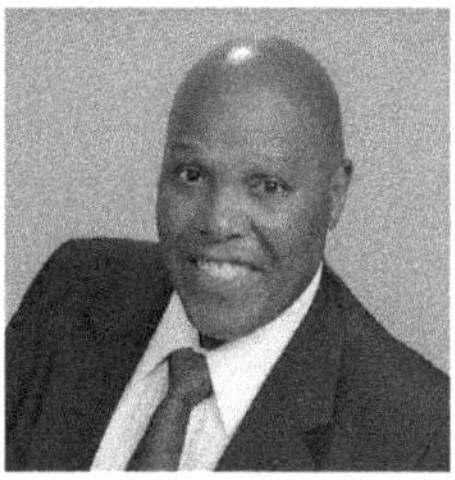

Rev. Duane Alfred Quamina is a writer, minister, and advocate whose work sits at the intersection of faith, health, and personal transformation.

Born on April 13, 1959, in Rochester, New York, his life has been shaped by a journey that spans adversity, self-discovery, and spiritual awakening. Through lived experience, disciplined study, and a commitment to truth, he has developed a perspective that challenges conventional thinking and calls individuals back to foundational principles.

As the founder of I Have A Dream Home, the Nonviolent Leadership Academy, and Project C.H.A.N.G.E. Masterclass Edition, Rev. Quamina teaches the practical application of spiritual principles in everyday life, with a focus on aligning the individual with systems that promote growth, stability, and long-term well-being.

In *Food For Thought*, he brings together scripture, observation, and modern research to explore a simple but often overlooked question: what did God originally intend for humanity to consume, and how does that design relate to the condition of the human body today?

His work is not driven by theory alone, but by experience—both observed and lived—and a desire to share what has the potential to restore clarity, health, and direction.

This book is part of a larger body of work aimed at encouraging individuals, families, and communities to think differently, live intentionally, and return to principles that sustain life.

EXPANDED SERIES

Food For Thought: Biblical Truths They Never Taught Us is a five-volume series exploring the relationship between scripture, health, and modern systems.

Volume 1: God's Original Diet and the Healing of the Nations
Explores God's original design for food and its connection to health.

Volume 2: Disease, Diet & Deception
Examines how modern dietary systems contribute to chronic disease.

Volume 3: Pharma vs. Prevention
Explores the contrast between medical dependency and natural prevention.

Volume 4: The Body as a Temple
Provides practical guidance for daily living and discipline.

Volume 5: Economic Systems of Food & Control
Examines how food systems shape availability, access, and community outcomes.

This series is not just information; it's structured progression:

- Truth
- Awareness
- Decision
- Discipline
- Structure

It is an invitation to reconsider what has been accepted as normal... and to move toward a more informed, intentional way of living.

NOTES & PERSONAL REFLECTIONS (PAGE 1)

NOTES & PERSONAL REFLECTIONS (PAGE 2)

NOTES & PERSONAL REFLECTIONS (PAGE 3)

www.ingramcontent.com/pod-product-compliance
Lightning Source LLC
LaVergne TN
LVHW050939210926
848482LV00013B/679
* 9 7 9 8 9 9 5 7 2 7 1 0 1 *